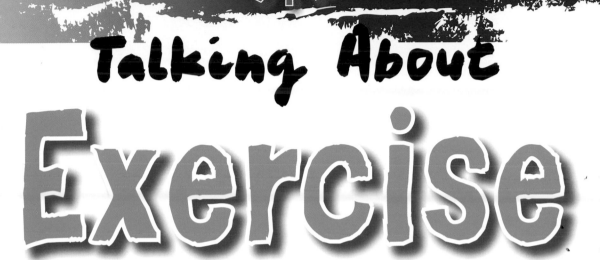

HEALTHY·LIVING

Talking About

Exercise

By Wendy St. Germain

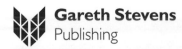

Gareth Stevens
Publishing

Please visit our Web site **www.garethstevens.com**. For a free color catalog of all our high-quality books, call toll free 1-800-542-2595 or fax 1-877-542-2596.

Library of Congress Cataloging-in-Publication Data

St. Germain, Wendy.
Talking about exercise / Wendy St Germain.
   p. cm. — (Healthy living)   Includes index.
 ISBN 978-1-4339-3662-3 (library binding)
 1. Exercise. 2. Physical fitness. I. Title.
 GV481.S666 2010
 613.7'1—dc22

                                   2009043441

Published in 2010 by
Gareth Stevens Publishing
111 East 14th Street, Suite 349
New York, NY 10003

© 2010 Blake Publishing

For Gareth Stevens Publishing:
Art Direction: Haley Harasymiw
Editorial Direction: Kerri O'Donnell

Cover photo: iStockphoto

Photos and illustrations: 0353
Dillon Naylor, pages 8 and 12; iStockphoto, pages 4–5, 8–9, 13 (bottom)–14, 16 (top)–17, 21 (bottom right)–22, 24–27; Photos.com, pages 5 (top right), 10–13, 15–16 (bottom), 18–21, 23, 25 (left)–26 (bottom right), 28–29, 30; UC Publishing, pages 5 (bottom left), 6, 9 (lower).

Printed in the United States of America

CPSIA compliance information: Batch #CW10GS: For further information contact Gareth Stevens, New York, New York, at 1-800-542-2595.

CONTENTS

Why do you need a healthy diet and exercise?......................4

What happens to your breathing when you exercise?...........6

How the heart works 8

Pulse..10

How everything works together 12

Body temperature...14

Thirst...16

Skin...18

Muscles..20

Muscular strength 22

Endurance and flexibility...24

Cold...26

Physical activity improves your health 28

It's never too late or too early to start!.......................30

Glossary 31

For Further Information and Index 32

Why do you need a healthy diet and exercise?

There are many reasons why you need a healthy diet and exercise. These things help you maintain strong bones, good muscle tone, and flexible joints. Even your mind benefits! Some people say you will stay smarter for longer by exercising and eating a healthy diet.

Do you want to be fit, healthy, and mentally active? Then be physically active. Your physical activity needs to include exercise that makes your heart work harder. Of course, walking, swimming, and other physical activity are not enough by themselves. You also need to eat healthy food to maintain your energy levels.

Without exercise, muscles shrink and get flabby. Because flabby muscles are not strong, they tire easily. Muscles keep your gut from sagging and your lungs working. Muscles make heat that keeps you warm. If you leap, bend, or reach, this is a result of a muscle action. Who wants weak and tired muscles when they are responsible for your body's every move?

Did you know?

With all the entertainment of computers, television, and electronic games, it is easy to forget to exercise. There are also many labor-saving devices to help us do our work. In today's world, you need to exercise more than ever. Without regular exercise, you use less than 10 percent of your muscles every day. People who spend long periods in front of the television or computer use even less!

Active lifestyles promote healthy, happy minds. Physically active people who eat a healthy diet learn more effectively. They also sleep and feel better.

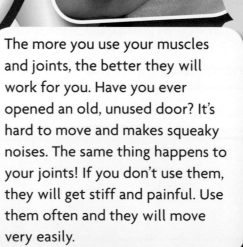

The more you use your muscles and joints, the better they will work for you. Have you ever opened an old, unused door? It's hard to move and makes squeaky noises. The same thing happens to your joints! If you don't use them, they will get stiff and painful. Use them often and they will move very easily.

There are many reasons why you need a healthy diet and exercise.

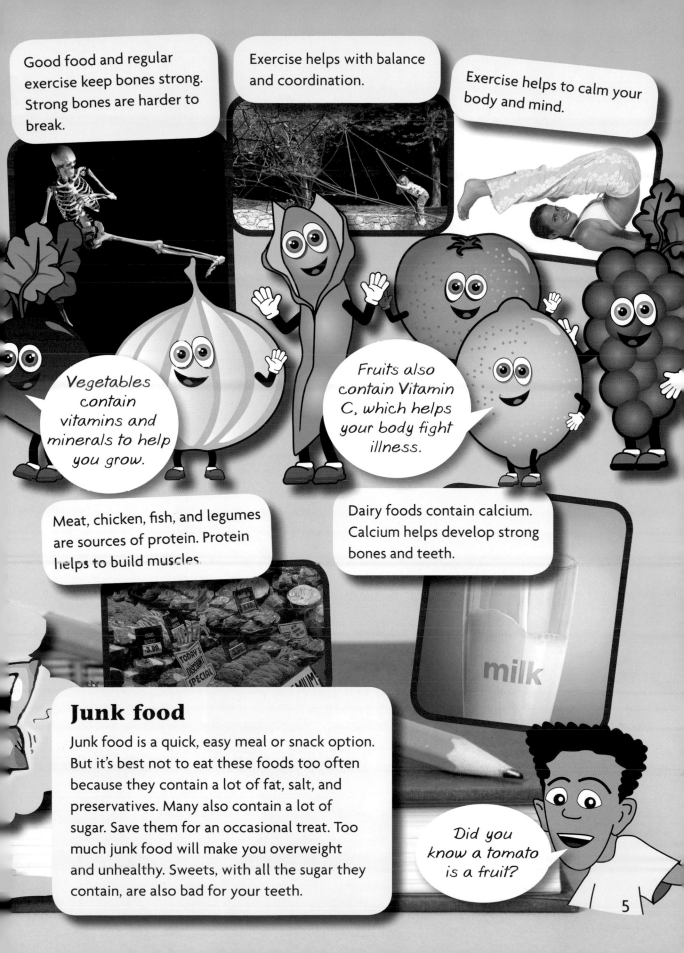

Good food and regular exercise keep bones strong. Strong bones are harder to break.

Exercise helps with balance and coordination.

Exercise helps to calm your body and mind.

Vegetables contain vitamins and minerals to help you grow.

Fruits also contain Vitamin C, which helps your body fight illness.

Meat, chicken, fish, and legumes are sources of protein. Protein helps to build muscles.

Dairy foods contain calcium. Calcium helps develop strong bones and teeth.

milk

Junk food

Junk food is a quick, easy meal or snack option. But it's best not to eat these foods too often because they contain a lot of fat, salt, and preservatives. Many also contain a lot of sugar. Save them for an occasional treat. Too much junk food will make you overweight and unhealthy. Sweets, with all the sugar they contain, are also bad for your teeth.

Did you know a tomato is a fruit?

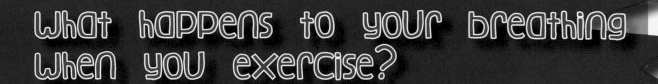

Our bodies are like cars. The faster they move, the more fuel they need to keep up the pace. The more briskly we exercise, the more energy and oxygen our muscles use.

Oxygen is delivered to your body **cells** by your blood. It usually takes about 20 seconds for an oxygen-rich, red blood cell to leave the heart and **circulate** throughout the whole body.

When you are exercising, oxygen must be delivered to your cells faster than usual. Cells demand more oxygen when working hard.

You have to breathe faster when you exercise. Every time you breathe in, you collect more oxygen for your blood. The faster you breathe in, the more oxygen you collect. The faster you breathe out, the more carbon dioxide you release.

oxygen

Get ready, lungs, I'm about to run!

6

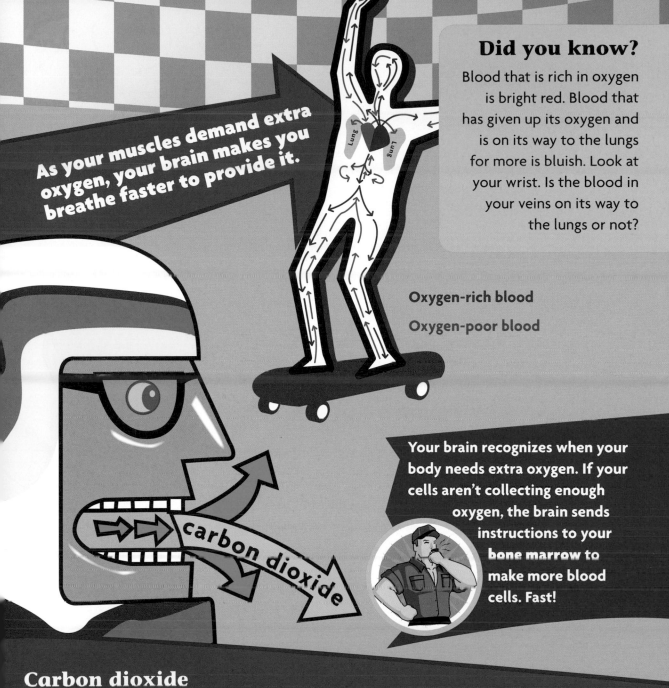

As your muscles demand extra oxygen, your brain makes you breathe faster to provide it.

Did you know?

Blood that is rich in oxygen is bright red. Blood that has given up its oxygen and is on its way to the lungs for more is bluish. Look at your wrist. Is the blood in your veins on its way to the lungs or not?

Oxygen-rich blood

Oxygen-poor blood

Your brain recognizes when your body needs extra oxygen. If your cells aren't collecting enough oxygen, the brain sends instructions to your **bone marrow** to make more blood cells. Fast!

carbon dioxide

Carbon dioxide

Humans are carbon-based creatures. Your foods have carbon **molecules** in them. Your body breaks these carbon molecules apart, removes the energy that holds them together, and uses that energy to run your body each day.

As part of this process, your cells combine single atoms of carbon with two atoms of oxygen to make carbon dioxide. You breathe out carbon dioxide as a waste product. Your body absolutely HAS to get rid of this carbon dioxide, so carbon dioxide is the main trigger to keep you breathing.

How the heart works

The heart is an organ. An organ is a group of tissues that work together to perform a certain function. Your heart is made up of many heart-muscle cells. Your heart delivers blood throughout your body, so it is important to keep it healthy.

One half of your heart sends oxygen-rich blood to your brain and the rest of your body. The other half of your heart collects blood that has delivered its oxygen and exchanged it for molecules of carbon dioxide. The harder you exercise, the faster this happens.

Your body demands more oxygen when you exercise, so your brain sends a message to your heart to pump faster. Exercise also produces more waste in the blood, so that must be quickly removed, too. The heart's job is to send blood around your body at the rate at which it is needed.

Did you know?
Your heart is about the same size as your fist.

Heart rate

Your blood vessels are elastic—they can stretch under pressure.

Every time your heart muscle contracts (tightens up and squeezes the blood out), it puts your blood vessels under pressure.

Between contractions (or beats), your heart relaxes and has a short rest. Like any other motor, it needs to rest or it will burn out. If you overexercise, your heart can suffer. Some symptoms include cramping, nausea, and feeling light-headed.

Keep your heart healthy

It is important to keep your heart healthy, and exercise helps do this. A well-exercised body means a well-exercised heart that works more effectively.

Like the rest of your body, your heart also needs a regular, fresh supply of blood. If your **arteries** are clogged with fat, the heart receives less blood. As you get older, your arteries can narrow, leading to heart disease. Heart disease can cause a heart attack, which leaves part of the heart muscle permanently damaged and unable to function.

Regular exercise helps reduce the risk of heart disease by keeping your arteries free of fatty deposits. Over time, some hardening of the arteries occurs naturally. However, with a good diet and regular exercise, this doesn't have to become a problem for your heart.

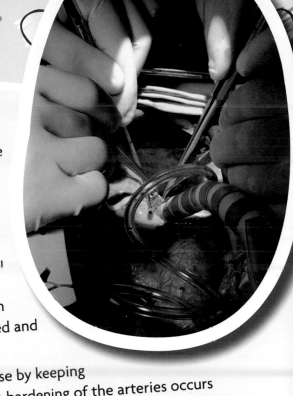

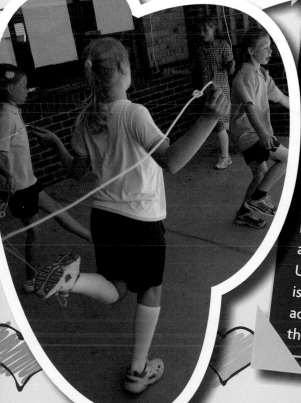

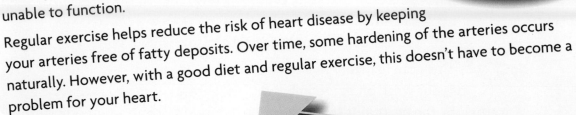

Jump Rope for Heart Health

The Jump Rope for Heart program began in the United States. The American Heart Association began the program over 30 years ago. Jump Rope for Heart is a national fundraising event for elementary school students. It promotes physical activity to help children learn the importance of exercise in building strong, healthy bodies. The program also teaches about helping others. Since Jump Rope for Heart began, more than $700 million have been raised for heart research and treatment. Millions of students across the United States take part. Jump Rope for Heart is also in other countries, promoting physical activity and heart-healthy living throughout the world.

PULSe

Squeeze and relax your fist a few times to see how contractions work. Heart contractions are called beats. You can count your heartbeats by taking your pulse.

You can feel your pulse by resting two fingers on the inside of your wrist, on the thumb side. That gentle throb you feel is caused by the heart as it sends oxygen-rich blood through your body.

When you exercise, your pulse throbs faster. The increase in speed comes from the heart pumping harder to meet your body's exercise needs. Light exercise increases heart rate (and therefore pulse) much less than intense exercise does. The harder you work, the harder your heart works.

Your weight, age, and even your sex will affect your pulse. For example, males tend to have larger bones than females of the same age, and the extra bone mass increases their weight. The more weight you carry, the more your heart must work to accommodate you.

Why is the nurse looking at her watch?

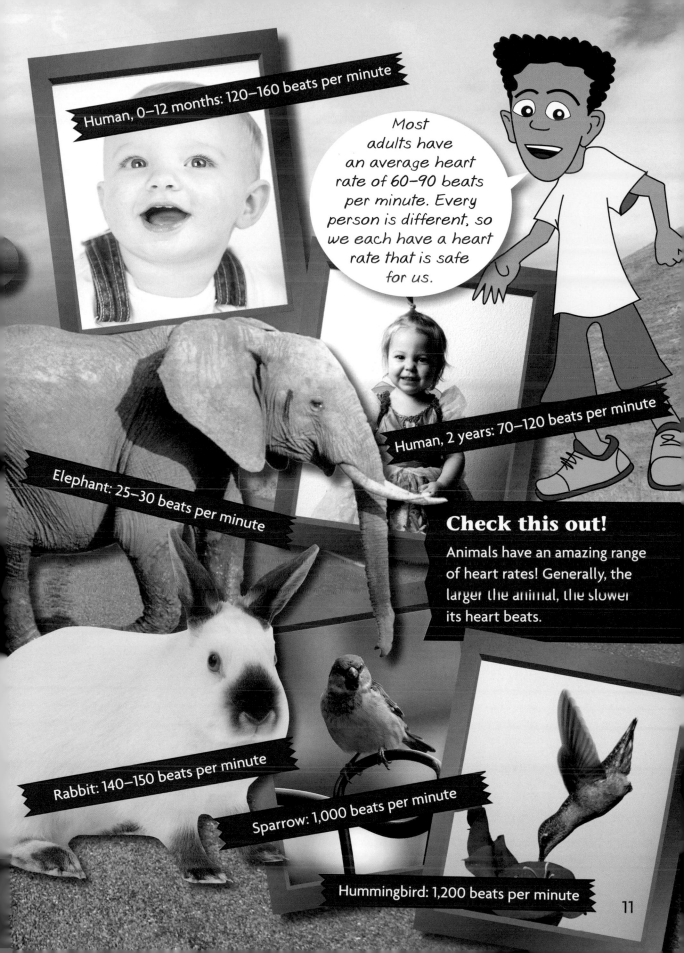

Human, 0–12 months: 120–160 beats per minute

Most adults have an average heart rate of 60–90 beats per minute. Every person is different, so we each have a heart rate that is safe for us.

Human, 2 years: 70–120 beats per minute

Elephant: 25–30 beats per minute

Check this out!

Animals have an amazing range of heart rates! Generally, the larger the animal, the slower its heart beats.

Rabbit: 140–150 beats per minute

Sparrow: 1,000 beats per minute

Hummingbird: 1,200 beats per minute

11

The cardiovascular system

Your **cardiovascular system** is made up of your heart and blood vessels (through which the blood travels). This system is like a highway for blood cells to travel along. While traveling, they deliver oxygen and nutrients throughout your body.

After your blood cells deliver the oxygen to wherever it is needed, they collect a molecule of carbon dioxide in its place. Carbon dioxide must not **accumulate** in our bodies. The blood carrying the carbon dioxide arrives in one side of the heart. The carbon dioxide is then delivered to the lungs, and every time we breathe out, our lungs send it into the air around us.

The word "cardio" comes from an old Latin word meaning "heart." "Vascular" means "vessels" (containers).

All things, including the tiny cells in your body, are made up of atoms and molecules. Atoms are tiny particles.

Molecules are made up of two or more atoms.

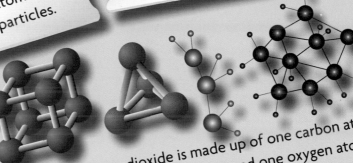

Oxygen is made up of two oxygen atoms. Carbon dioxide is made up of one carbon atom and two oxygen atoms. Water is made up of two hydrogen atoms and one oxygen atom.

Red blood cells are formed in bone marrow. These cells carry oxygen around your body and remove carbon dioxide. If they are not damaged, they last about 120 days.

Damaged cells are gobbled up by special cells whose job is to keep the bloodstream clean.

Old cells make their way to two important organs, the liver and the spleen. Here, they are destroyed. Without this constant creation of new blood cells and destruction of old or damaged ones, our bodies would soon be starved of oxygen and carbon dioxide would build up. We would not survive!

People breathe in oxygen.

People breathe out carbon dioxide.

Trees and plants love carbon dioxide. They '"breathe" it in. In exchange, they "breathe" out the oxygen we need. Every time we breathe in, we take fresh oxygen into our lungs. This oxygen is collected by our blood cells and delivered back to the side of the heart that sends it through the body.

Body temperature

Physical activity uses your muscles and heats up your body. Your body must be kept at a steady temperature of 98.6° F (37°C).

Working muscles need more oxygen than resting muscles and need to remove carbon dioxide faster. How long and hard you exercise affects how quickly you heat up.

Hot and bothered

The faster your blood circulates, the faster oxygen is delivered and carbon dioxide is removed. However, when you exercise hard, you will soon find yourself red in the face, as well as having red blotches all over you. This is your body bringing heated blood to the surface to cool. Luckily, most healthy people tend to run out of breath before the heart is placed at risk of being overworked.

You might wonder why, if you are only exercising certain muscles, your whole body heats up. Well, it's a good thing it does!

Muscles are made of protein fibers. Proteins are easily damaged or destroyed when overheated. Your brain detects the change in body temperature and knows that the working muscles cannot be allowed to overheat. To prevent this, excess heat is shared with the rest of the body.

Heat causes the body to lose fluid. When the amount of body fluid drops too low, **dehydration** occurs.

In extreme heat conditions, the human body can lose up to 0.8 gallons (3 l) of fluid per hour!

Overheating

Temperature also affects how your body reacts. During hot months, outdoor exercise is best done in the cooler morning and evening hours.

Overheating (**heatstroke**), if untreated, can lead to brain, kidney, or liver damage, and even death. Heatstroke symptoms include headache, nausea, cramping, exhaustion, and unconsciousness. Heat stress is a milder form of overheating and happens to many people in warm weather. You don't have to exercise for long to experience heat stress.

Whether you exercise or not, drink plenty of fluids (water and unsweetened fruit juice are better than sugary drinks) when it's hot. Stay in the shade when possible. If you feel ill, drink fluids, find a cool area, and take a cool shower or wipe yourself with a cool cloth if you can. If you don't improve, see your doctor.

Why we sweat

Have you ever been sprayed with mist on a hot day? It cools you down! Sweat works the same way. **Sweat glands** release moisture all over your body. The average person has over 2.5 million sweat glands.

Sweat is a watery solution that contains salt and other substances. If you lick your skin after you sweat, you'll taste the saltiness. That salt was flushed from your body when you were sweating!

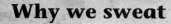

You sweat all the time, but it's only when you feel hot that you notice.

As you heat up during exercise, tiny **capillaries** bring the blood to the surface to release heat through the skin. This causes red, blotchy marks. They disappear after you cool down.

Why do you get hot when you have a fever?

Fever is your body's way of fighting infection. Many germs that make you sick can't survive high temperatures, so fever destroys them. Since exercise also heats you up, it's dangerous to exercise when you have a fever.

Many dogs also suffer heat stress if exercised during peak hours. Remember, they're wearing fur coats!

Your body can absorb too much heat from the sun. If you can't cool down fast enough, this external heat can also be dangerous.

About 75 percent of the human body is made up of water. If you weigh 110 pounds (50 kg), about 77 pounds (35 kg) is water! Water keeps your body temperature steady. If it turns cold when you are at the beach, dip your finger in the sea. The water will be warm because it doesn't change its temperature as fast as the air does.

WATER KEEPS CELLS FROM DRYING OUT. MANY THINGS NEED TO BE DISSOLVED IN WATER TO KEEP THE BODY HEALTHY. WATER MIXES WITH TINY PARTICLES IN OUR BODY. IT ALSO CARRIES WASTE AWAY. WHEN YOU EXERCISE, YOUR CELLS NEED MORE FLUID TO KEEP UP WITH NORMAL BODY PROCESSES, WHICH MOVE FASTER TO DEAL WITH THE DEMANDS OF EXERCISE.

Cells and water

When cells don't have enough water, they shrink and can become brittle.

It's important to drink plenty of water every day, especially on hot days. You can't always tell when your cells are losing water. Coffee, tea, and sodas (and some "power drinks") can increase dehydration. If you don't like drinking lots of water, try freezing water into ice cubes and suck on those. You can also eat watermelon and other watery fruits.

Exercise increases your **metabolism** and your body's demand for fluid. In order for your body to perform its usual tasks and keep up with the heat you produce while exercising, drinking more fluids is important.

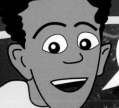

Every living thing needs water.

Sports drinks

Athletes who undertake long periods of exercise often refuel with sports drinks to recover from the workout. These drinks **replenish** fluids, minerals, and electrolytes (important in chemical reactions) that are lost during the work-out.

Some people worry about sports drinks making you fat because they contain sugar. They are best used by people who have had an energetic workout of about 40 minutes or more. Without exercise, sports drinks can have the same effect as any other sugared drink.

Your brain notices when your body loses more water than it takes in. This often happens when you exercise.

Water is lost first from the spaces between your cells. Your brain sends messages to your cells to find water. If you don't replace the lost water by drinking, your cells will be the next to lose it. Fluid lost from muscle tissue can cause cramping.

By the time you feel thirsty, your cells need a drink. When your head aches from the heat and dehydration, that's your brain trying very hard to make you notice how thirsty your cells are.

Some common signs of dehydration are:

• headache, dizziness

• dry lips and mouth

• thirst (but if you are too dehydrated, your thirst trigger can actually shut down)

• stomach and muscle cramping

• feeling weak and tired

• little or no urine when you go to the bathroom

Rather than having one big drink before exercising, it's better to drink a small amount of water and then sip it regularly throughout your workout. Keep refueling those cells at a steady pace. Have a few mouthfuls about every 15 minutes.

Did you know?

Urine can give clues to whether you are dehydrated. Pale urine suggests you are well hydrated. Urine the color of apple juice or darker suggests you are dehydrated.

SKIN

Swimming is fun and an excellent way to exercise. It works just about every muscle in your body. It expands your lungs, increasing the amount of oxygen you can take in (and carbon dioxide you can release).

By swimming in cool water, the risk of overheating is reduced, especially if you are in a shaded area. But just as sun **exposure** can cause skin damage, swimming pools can cause problems, too.

Swimming pools must be kept as clean as possible. Unfortunately, the chemicals used to disinfect pools can cause problems, though the problems caused by swimming in water not disinfected would be far worse.

Chlorine

Chlorine is the most commonly used pool disinfectant. People with sensitive skin often suffer from swimming in **chlorinated** water—especially if too much chlorine has been used. Chlorinated water can cause rashes, eczema, and irritations to the eyes, nose, and mouth.

Lifeguards and other people who spend a lot of time in and around pools often experience problems. Persistent colds, eye irritations, and headaches are some of the more common complaints, particularly in indoor pools. This is because chlorine gas can build up if the pool area isn't well **ventilated**.

Skin doesn't absorb chlorine. But if chlorine fumes come into contact with the lining of the nose and mouth and the delicate eye tissue, they can react to form an acid that burns. When blood vessels in the ear, nose, and throat become irritated, they can swell, leading to reduced oxygen circulation and pressure on tissues. The brain sends a message that things aren't quite right. The message is often a headache.

Once you leave the pool area and return to fresh air, the blood vessels should shrink back to normal size.

Be sure to shower after you swim. By rinsing off the chlorinated water, you reduce the effects it might have on your skin. Applying a light moisturizer will also help fight the drying effects of the chlorinated water.

Sun protection

Remember, if you're swimming outside in a pool or at the beach, use sunscreen—and if possible, a UV swimsuit! As well as the rays shining directly down on you, the sun reflects off the water and onto your skin. This increases the severity of the sunburn you might experience.

muscles

The more exercise we do, the stronger our bodies become. Regular exercise strengthens your bones and muscles. Like a good diet, exercise helps you to grow big and strong.

Every time you exercise, muscle-growing activities are triggered. If you exercise every day, you will become a bit stronger each day. You won't notice the little changes each day, but if you look at a photograph of yourself after a few months, you will see how exercise has led to muscle growth.

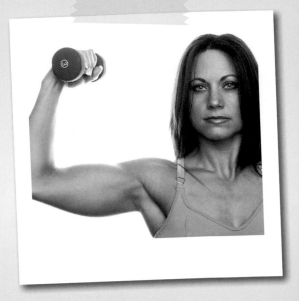

Muscle growth

Muscle growth is a complicated process. Regular exercise triggers the production of growth hormones. Some of these hormones help grow muscle tissue. Others work on bones or other body parts. The muscle fibers grow both in size and number of new protein fibers that can be added to existing muscle.

Males grow bigger muscles because they produce a special hormone called **testosterone**. One of its jobs is to promote muscle growth.

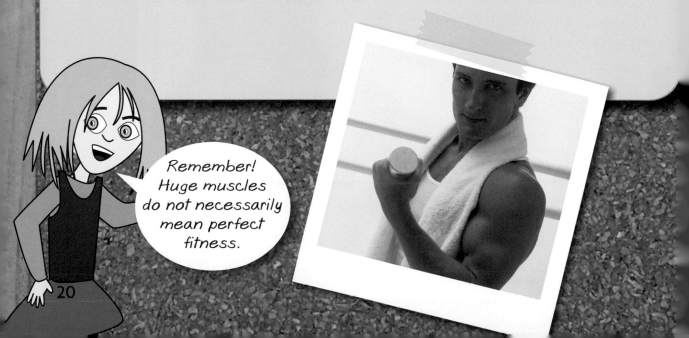

Remember! Huge muscles do not necessarily mean perfect fitness.

20

Strong bodies have great endurance!

Trained athletes and sports people did not get their strength and **endurance** overnight! They had to work at it gradually.

The greater your endurance, the less easily you become tired.

8, 9, 10 ...

You must never rush fitness training. You might damage your body. Take time. Do it in steps.

Some people build up their bodies by using **steroids** or other drugs. It is illegal and dangerous to use the drugs for this purpose.

It is also worth remembering that building your strength will not improve your flexibility.

Exercise fuel

To exercise, you need fuel. Protein, fats, and **carbohydrates** are all good fuels for exercise. Carbohydrates are the best fuels to provide quick energy. It is important to have all three of these types of fuels in your diet.

About 30 minutes before exercise, have a small carbohydrate snack. This will provide you with extra energy.

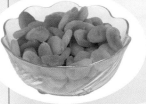

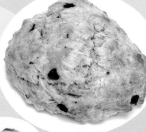

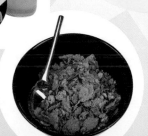

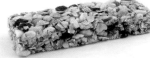

muscular strength

Your heart is a muscle—just like all the muscles that allow you to walk, breathe, move, and speak.

A muscle must be able to quickly create the force required to move an object (and change its direction). This force requires short bursts of energy. This energy is called muscular strength.

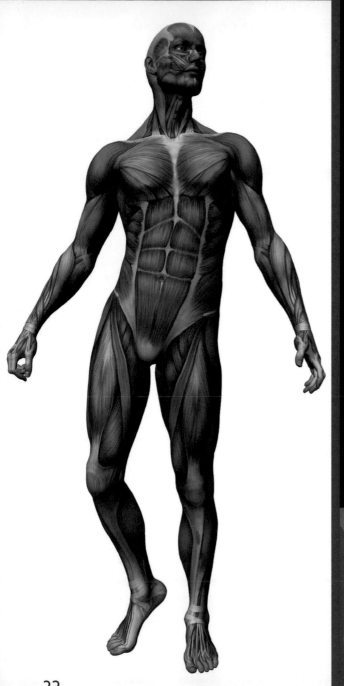

Muscular strength describes the strength your muscles can endure, how much they can "manage."

Muscles provide physical strength, the power you have to do tasks, and your ability to do them over a period of time. Strong muscles can endure more. Working your muscles helps them to grow, but remember, they need fluids to recover after the workout.

Tissues are groups of similar cells that work together to do a special job.

Study the fibers that make up your clothes and see how they fit together lengthwise. Muscle tissue is assembled in a similar, strandlike way. It lies in rows, a bit like uncooked spaghetti in a package! The strands of muscle fiber form bundles that work together. These bundles are called muscles.

A steak is an example of animal muscle tissue.

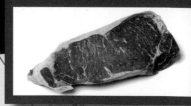

22

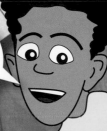

The word "strength" comes from an old English word meaning "strong."

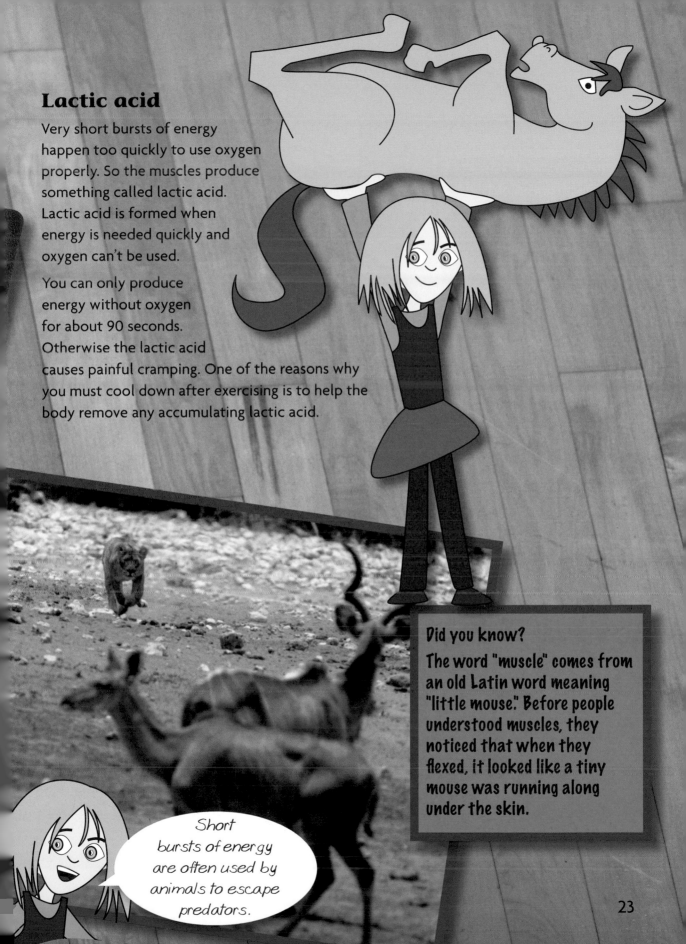

Lactic acid

Very short bursts of energy happen too quickly to use oxygen properly. So the muscles produce something called lactic acid. Lactic acid is formed when energy is needed quickly and oxygen can't be used.

You can only produce energy without oxygen for about 90 seconds. Otherwise the lactic acid causes painful cramping. One of the reasons why you must cool down after exercising is to help the body remove any accumulating lactic acid.

Did you know?
The word "muscle" comes from an old Latin word meaning "little mouse." Before people understood muscles, they noticed that when they flexed, it looked like a tiny mouse was running along under the skin.

Short bursts of energy are often used by animals to escape predators.

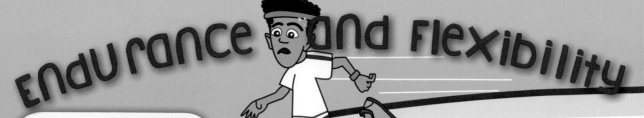

Endurance and Flexibility

The word "endurance" comes from an old Latin word meaning "to harden or strengthen."

"Endurance" means continuing when things get difficult.

Physical endurance is your ability to keep doing something that requires strength and energy. Endurance exercise doesn't always look hard, but you need a strong and fit body to do it. All-day walks and long-distance cycling races might look easy, but the people involved must be in peak physical condition to perform the tasks without injuring themselves.

While you are alive, your heart constantly beats. This is an example of endurance.

Flexibility

It is important that your muscles and tendons can stretch. This is called flexibility.

Flexibility is an important part of being able to move.

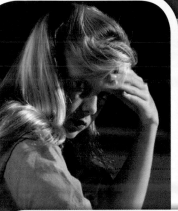

Endurance can be emotional and mental as well as physical. Emotional endurance means how long you can keep doing something that is not easy for you. Mental endurance is your ability to keep going when you want to quit. It is not always easy to keep your mind focused on the task you are doing. Mental endurance is about not giving up, even when things get tough.

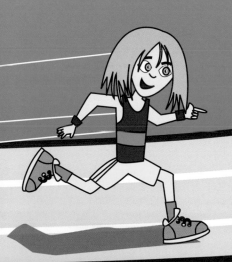

A properly trained athlete has great physical and mental endurance. Usually you need both to become really good at a sport.

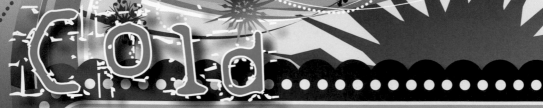

Cold

When your body temperature drops, your blood flow slows. Your blood vessels get smaller (constrict). This conserves more heat for your body. That's why you turn blue if you are very cold. The blood vessels have shrunk, and there's less red blood going to your skin. Oxygen doesn't reach your cells as quickly, and waste products are removed more slowly.

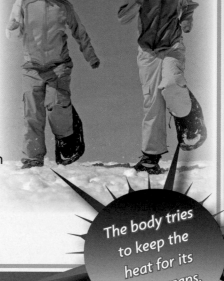

Since we need more oxygen circulating when we exercise (and faster waste removal), it is important to take care when exercising in cold weather.

The parts of your body farthest from your heart are the first to suffer from cold.

> The body tries to keep the heat for its vital organs.

What is a shiver?

A shiver is your body's attempt to warm your muscles. It does this by causing them to tighten (contract) and relax over and over. This gives each muscle a tiny warm-up.

Shivering causes goose bumps. Goose bumps get their name because little bumps rise on your skin, making it look much like a plucked goose! Raising the skin causes the hairs on it to stand up. This acts like a tiny blanket, holding any warmth your body is giving off close to you. (The opposite happens when you are too hot, allowing the warm air to escape.)

> Many activities occur in cold weather. Cold can be just as dangerous to the body as overheating.

Be aware that if you are shivering while you exercise outside, your body is telling you it is suffering cold exposure and needs to be warmed up. Find somewhere warm and have a warm drink or bowl of soup.

Exposure to cold air can slow down your body's **immune system**. This is why getting chilled can sometimes lead to cold or flu.

Frostbite occurs when the outer layer of skin freezes. This often leaves purplish marks.

When exercising in cold weather, remember to do the following:

◆ Wear layers. Layers produce little pockets of warmth that are more effective at keeping the body warm than one thick layer is.

◆ Keep all body parts dry.

◆ Keep your head warm—wear a hat.

◆ Cover your mouth with a scarf to help warm the air you are taking into your lungs.

◆ Slow down and cool off a little if you feel yourself overheating. Remember, your body will be heating up as you exercise. Even if it's cold outside, your insides can heat up.

◆ Keep drinking fluids. Just because it's not hot doesn't mean you can't become dehydrated!

Many people make the mistake of thinking that you only need to drink fluids when exercising in warm weather. It is just as important to keep drinking fluids in ALL weather! Bodies can overheat in cold weather, too.

Physical activity improves your health

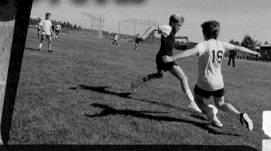

Overall health comes from a healthy immune system, strong muscles, and a body that is properly cared for. Here are some of the ways regular physical activity keeps you healthy and increases your energy levels.

Controlling your weight

Exercise burns fat. Regular exercise helps keep your weight at a healthy level. With a healthy diet, your body will use its stores of fat to fuel exercise. Once the fat stores are used up, if you continue to eat a healthy diet and keep up the exercise, the fat won't return!

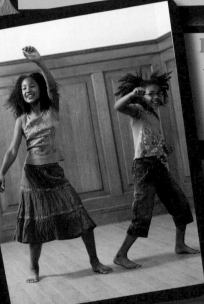

Improving learning and memory

Your brain works best with a combination of rest, good diet, and a good oxygen supply. Good blood flow, resulting from regular exercise, means the brain gets the oxygen it needs.

Keeping your heart healthy

Regular exercise keeps the heart muscle strong. Exercise helps to keep blood pressure at a healthy level, meaning that between beats the heart gets a proper rest. For people with high blood pressure, the heart doesn't fully rest between beats. This can lead to a heart attack.

Helping reduce effects of allergies and asthma

A healthy immune system can cope better with pollens than a weak one can. Exercise helps people with asthma, too. It expands the air passages, allowing more oxygen to enter the lungs. Swimming is excellent exercise for people with asthma. Physical activity regulates breathing. For people with asthma (who have irregular breathing patterns), this can make a big difference in the amount of oxygen they take in.

Building stronger joints and muscles

Muscles and joints work better if they are exercised. Tendons, ligaments, and muscles grow stronger with exercise. They also become more flexible. Stronger joints and muscles are also harder to injure and tend to recover more quickly if injury occurs.

Reducing headaches

Regular exercise when you are feeling well can reduce the severity of some headaches when they do come. It can even prevent new headaches. Exercise can produce certain pain-killing (and mood-improving) chemical substances. If you have recurring headaches, be sure to see your doctor.

Reducing your cholesterol

Regular exercise helps to break up the deposits of bad **cholesterol** that can build up in your circulatory system, clogging your arteries. Cholesterol sticks to the sides of the artery and can harden, making the area through which blood flows narrower.

Helping you sleep better

A well-exercised body can appreciate rest time. Exercise reduces (or even eliminates) muscle stress. An unstressed muscle can relax better. Clench your fist, then relax it. Which felt more relaxing—the clenched (stressed) muscle or the resting one?

Reducing depression and anxiety

People who are fit tend to suffer less depression and anxiety. When you feel nervous or anxious, certain chemical substances are produced by the body. A buildup of these substances can make your negative mood even worse. Exercise reduces the levels of these substances by carrying them away with the rest of the waste your body accumulates. Exercise also produces substances that improve your mood. One good way to shake a bad mood is to do some exercise. (The vitamin D from sunshine also helps to improve the mood, but remember to wear sunscreen and a hat.)

It's never too late or too early to start!

Many people think that you have to start exercising when you are young. It's best if you do, but many older people can tell you they have also benefited from exercise programs.

Exercise helps you to maintain your balance. In older people, this is very important because they often fall as a result of poor balance.

With regular exercise for the rest of your life, you will keep your heart and lungs strong. You won't feel the same stiffness in your joints that many others feel as they age.

Physical activity keeps your muscles flexible. Strong, flexible muscles keep their shape and work well.

A well-exercised body regularly keeps in touch with the brain and this, with strong muscles, is what helps to increase your reaction time.

Throughout your life, bones can benefit by physical activity:

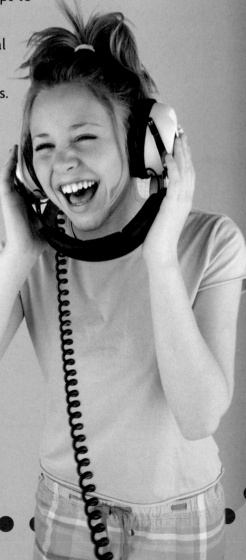

- When you're young, exercise builds strong bones. It's when you're young that you can reach the peak of your bone mass, so get as much as you can while you can!

- As you get older, exercise keeps bones strong and compacted.

- When you are old, your bones will be harder to break if you keep fit.

Regular exercise can add years to your life!

Did you know?
Singers need to warm up their vocal cords with a few practice notes to get them ready. Otherwise, they can strain their vocal cords just like a muscle can be strained.

GLOSSARY

accumulate	gradually increase the amount
arteries	largest of the tubes that carry blood from your heart to the rest of your body
bone marrow	the soft substance in the hollow center of bones
capillaries	the smallest type of blood vessels
carbohydrates	foods that provide the body with energy, such as rice, potatoes, and bread
cardiovascular system	the heart and the vessels through which the blood flows in your body
cells	the basic, functional parts of a living thing
chlorinated	having had chlorine (a disinfectant) added
chlorine	greenish-yellow gas with a strong smell, used to keep swimming pools clean
cholesterol	a chemical substance found in your blood
circulate	to flow throughout
dehydration	the loss of too much fluid from the body
endurance	the ability to keep doing something difficult over a long period of time
exposure	the harmful effects on your body of being outside in weather extremes
heatstroke	fever or weakness caused by being outside in the heat of the sun for too long
immune system	the system by which your body protects itself from disease
metabolism	the chemical process by which food is changed into energy in your body
molecules	units made of two or more atoms
replenish	to put new supplies into something
steroids	illegal drugs that enhance performance
sweat glands	small organs under your skin that produce sweat
testosterone	the hormone in males that gives them their male qualities
ventilated	open to let in fresh air

For Further Information

Books

Libal, Autumn. *The Importance of Physical Activity and Exercise: The Fitness Factor.* Broomall, PA: Mason Crest Publishers, 2005.

Schaefer, Adam. *Exercise.* Mankato, MN: Heinemann/Raintree Publishers, 2009.

Web Sites

Easy Fitness Activities for Kids

www.howstuffworks.com/easy-fitness-activities-for-kids.htm

Kidnetic.com

www.kidnetic.com

Index

arteries 9, 29

balance 5, 30

blood 6, 7, 8, 9, 10, 12, 13, 14, 15, 19, 26, 28, 29

bone marrow 7, 13

bones 4, 5, 10, 20, 30

brain 7, 8, 14, 17, 28, 30

breathing 6, 7, 13, 22, 28

calcium 5

carbohydrates 21

carbon dioxide 6, 7, 8, 12, 13, 14, 18

cardiovascular system 12

cells 6, 7, 8, 12, 13, 16, 17, 22, 26

chlorine 18, 19

cold 26, 27

coordination 5

dehydration 14, 16, 17, 27

diet 4, 9, 20, 28

endurance 21, 24, 25

exposure 18, 27

fever 15

flexibility 4, 21, 25, 29, 30

frostbite 27

goose bumps 26

heart 4, 6,, 8, 9, 10, 11, 12, 13, 14, 22, 24, 26, 28, 30

heart rate 8, 10, 11

heat 14, 15, 16, 27

joints 4, 29, 30

junk food 5

lungs 4, 6, 7, 12, 13, 18, 27, 28, 30

muscle growth 20

muscles 4, 5, 6, 7, 8, 9, 14, 17, 18, 20, 22, 23, 25, 26, 28, 29, 30

overheating 14, 18, 26, 27

oxygen 6, 7, 8, 10, 12, 13, 14, 18, 19, 23, 26, 28

pulse 10

shiver 26, 27

skin 18, 19, 26, 27

sports drinks 17

sunscreen 19

sweat 15

thirst 17

urine 17